Simply Skin

Learn How to Improve the Health and Appearance of your Skin

by Angela Freeman

Published in Great Britain by:

Angela Freeman
39 Compton Avenue
Brighton
East Sussex
BN1 3PT
United Kingdom

angelafreemanbooks@gmail.com

ISBN-13: {978-1986835220}
ISBN-10: {1986835227}

Table of Contents

Introduction

First of all, I wanted to commend you; on deciding to get the very best out of your skin. By taking personal action and utilising the knowledge from this book, you are firmly on the path to improving the health and appearance of your skin.

Nowadays, when you go into a beauty hall or online, you are surrounded by information on skincare. There is a vast array of products available, with a whole range of varying advice presented, often inaccurately explained, and out of context. This book will tell you truthfully, exactly what you want to know, concisely and without agenda. Guiding you through, step by step, on how you can personally achieve healthy clear skin.

Simply Skin is your own personal guide, giving you a solid understanding of what is affecting your skin and why. While providing you with accurate steps outlining how you can achieve healthy, clear, radiant skin. As the book unfolds, you will gain the knowledge and understanding behind this advice, so you can fully understand how your skin will benefit.

Your skin and its health and appearance are so intricately linked and influenced, that with the right guidance, maintenance and correct application of products, it can be dramatically altered to your advantage.

By following and applying a select number of key golden rules, devised by myself; which when applied together have had amazing success, and helped hundreds of my clients over the last 10 years, leaving them with the best skin they've ever had. This book will outline what truly makes **THE** difference between good skin and great skin and what it is you need to do.

Throughout this book I have carefully pre-empted and answered the most common questions which I have often been faced with over the years, stemming from poor advice or lack of knowledge. Putting any confusion finally to rest and outlining and debunking a lot of common misconceptions.

After identifying your individual skin type at the start of this book, you will notice references throughout; aimed to guide you through and provide you with tailored advice for your individual skin type. I will give you an accurate home routine you can follow and of course the 'Golden Rules' to achieve clear, healthy skin and maximise results.

As well as showing you how to carry out your own luxury facials at home and how to integrate these treatments into your lifestyle.

The second half of my book looks at the most common skin concerns affecting individuals:

• Darkness and Puffiness around the eyes

• Whiteheads, Blackheads & Acne

• Enlarged Pores

• Eczema/dermatitis

• Psoriasis

• Rosacea

• Age Spots/Dark Spots and Pigmentation

Each chapter outlines the most common causes and triggers to bring them about. Along with recommended accessible actions and treatments you can directly adopt and apply, to help fight the appearance of these common skin concerns. Including, topical application of products, home treatments, oral supplements and foods, and prevention techniques.

Although tempting to jump around please take my advice and take the time to read through the skincare and facial element from start to finish, it builds upon previous knowledge gained throughout the book, to give you the entire picture of what your skin needs, and as a result you, will gain so much more from it. Heaven forbid you also miss out on a golden rule! Then please head to any relevant skin concerns that you may be suffering from at present, or have had in the past, for recommended treatment and advice.

I discovered from a young age that my skin was very sensitive, prone to eczema and redness. My skin would flair up with redness, patches triggered in seconds by stress or the wrong ingredient. While at the same time if I didn't keep up a good skin routine, my combination skin would follow an extreme route with either severe dryness or congestion. So, I can truly say I can relate to a lot of skin concerns.

In my desire to bring out the best skin I could in me, I developed a passion for skin care, which extended past interest into a fulfilling career which has allowed me to pursue my passion and fixation in achieving healthy, clear, radiant skin. This book has allowed me to share all my knowledge from the last ten years, of what truly makes a difference to skin, allowing me to utilise all the thousands of conversations I've had on skin into one concise book. I wish there had been a personal guide out there like this, to help me when I needed it.

A dermatologist is not on the radar for the average person, so being able to treat your skin at home effectively is so important. I hope this book will not only guide you to look after and treat your skin effectively but also prevent you from spending money and emotions on solutions that don't work. Having done it myself, I understand how desperate you can get, and how upsetting it can be to find you've not been given the correct advice. I hope this guide will go a long way in preventing this scenario. I've spent the last decade of my life dedicating myself to learning all the secrets of the skin, studying training and expanding my knowledge, and applying this to my customers. The results achieved and feedback from my ladies and my male clients has been amazing. So, without further hesitation, I wish you the very best in your journey to 'great skin'.

With all my Love

Angela Freeman

Chapter 1:
What is skin and what does it do?

Skin is the body's largest organ; it is made up of three key layers:

The outermost layer is known as the **epidermis** (Ep-ih-DER-mis). This is the one that you scrub off when you exfoliate either your face or body. This layer is constantly shedding dead cells from its surface; with new skin cells surfacing from beneath to take their place.

Beneath this outer layer is the **dermis** (DER-mis). This contains blood vessels which oxygenate the skin.

While the deepest layer, the third layer, is called the **subcutis** (Sub-KEW-tis). This is where fat cells are stored to protect muscles and bones, providing a cushion of protection.

If you look very closely at your skin, you are likely to see small holes, these are known as pores and are visible all over the face and body. You will also notice hairs, these grow through from the dermis (the middle layer), up through the epidermis (the top layer). At the root of this hair, there are glands, which cause sweat and sebum. Sweat is designed to be a mechanism to cool us down and remove waste products and toxins from our body. While sebum, an oily substance, is designed to help us lock in moisture and trap bacteria.

The skin acts as a natural barrier of protection from the external environment, protecting us from various bacteria and microbes, chemicals, sunlight and other environmental factors.

Chapter 2:
How much of what we apply to the skin is absorbed into our bodies?

In one camp, we have those who say the skin is such an effective barrier that hardly anything will reach down to the deepest layers of the skin, let alone the bloodstream. While others say the complete opposite with claims on the internet stating that 64% of chemicals found in products are absorbed by our skin. So, who's right?

First of all, our skin is a very effective barrier; it is very difficult for chemicals to travel through all the layers of our skin, let alone into our bloodstream.

Mayonnaise

The very outer layer of the epidermis, (which is made up of sub-layers) known as the stratum corneum, is hydrophobic "water-hating". This is why we don't absorb all the water, swelling into a big balloon every time we have a bath or go swimming. Although water molecules do penetrate the skin, the skin's preference is lipophilic "oil-loving", this is the reason why oils penetrate deeper into the skin. Although oils themselves don't reach that much further down, because of the increase in water content the deeper down you go into the epidermis. The more water it contains, the harder it is for oil to penetrate. If you remember from school or even the last time you made a vinaigrette for your salad, oil and water repel each other. They separate and are unable to mix, with oil on the top trapping water beneath it. The same applies to our skin; this handy mechanism keeps moisture and hydration locked into our skin, so it doesn't dry out.

In fact, it is so hard for water and oil to penetrate our skin, skincare companies have had to come up with their own blend of mayonnaise. Because the barrier of oil and water works so effectively, creams have to be emulsified. Designed specifically to be amphiphilic (part oil and water) so products can reach slightly deeper into the skin to deliver said benefits.

The Vital Difference between Penetration and Absorption

Skin Penetration looks at the epidermis. The epidermis itself is made up of five layers. When you are talking about skin penetration, you are looking at the amount of topically applied chemical that can penetrate and exist from the top layer, (the outermost layer the stratum corneum) all the way through to the bottom layer (the stratum basale). During penetration, the body does not yet absorb the chemical, and it cannot affect the body systems. Skin care products are designed to be in this bracket.

Skin Absorption occurs when the topically applied chemical breaks the skin barrier to reach the bloodstream. The Food Drug Administration (FDA) or Medicine and Healthcare products Regulatory Agency (MHRA) specifically look at this, along with what happens after absorption. (Certain chemicals can react with enzymes, changing state, making them more toxic.) All of this is considered when approving skin care products for safety, preventing said products from being approved unless specifically designed for this purpose.

Generally speaking, should an unwanted chemical get absorbed into the body, our natural response is to filter out the chemical via bodily fluids (sweat, urine, excretion, etc.) preventing bioaccumulation (build up) occurring.

The Body's Natural Defence Mechanisms

Our bodies are on autopilot with various systems in place to help prevent penetration of foreign chemicals and bacteria. It's not necessarily easy to gain entry.

The Bodies way of preventing penetration:

•First, the size of the molecule is taken into account. If it is too big, it can't penetrate the skin. Some will fail at the first hurdle; others won't.

•Oil, produced by glands all over your body, has a tendency to trap bacteria on the skin, preventing them from getting any further.

•The skin itself is also covered with non-pathogenic bacteria or as I like to call them, 'good bacteria'. These compete with pathogenic micro-organisms, or 'bad bacteria', for nutrients and surface area of cells. This good bacteria naturally produces anti-bacterial proteins that prevent colonisation of the bad bacteria.

•Our epithelial cells, whether on the surface of the skin or lining our organs, also produce chemical substances that are micro-biocidal which kill bacteria or inhibit their growth. In fact, we have enzymes in our sweat and antibacterial peptides in our skin constantly working to fight bacteria.

•Should it gain entry, the composition of the chemical is taken into account; is it soluble? This will affect how far it can penetrate.

•Also, the area of the body that the chemicals have contact with will increase or decrease the success rate. Some areas of the body have more layers of skin, such as the palms of the hands and soles of the feet, which makes penetration a lot harder.

•Those that do penetrate will come in contact with our enzymes, especially adept at recognising pathogens. These enzymes are designed to break down any foreign toxic chemicals and deactivate them. After entering tissues, pathogens are recognised, ingested and killed by phagocytes. A very significant and effective defence mechanism.

•Your body then constantly regulates and filters out any unwanted chemicals via sweat, urine, etc.

Conclusion

This is where perspective is needed; there is a big difference between micro-analysing a pot of face cream and a bottle of bleach how they would affect the skin.

So, I'm going to say, claims such as '64% of all chemicals are absorbed into our skin' are biased and not a true, accurate representation of what happens with our skin. This has put a spin on absorption rates which has worried a lot of people, I've had women coming up to me in distress stating these claims, so I would like to put your mind at ease. There are always ways for chemicals to make it into our blood system. Our skin is not impermeable; we are not made of glass. There will be some molecules that make it into the deepest layers of the skin where our blood vessels are. Your body has a great way of defending itself, called to action automatically whenever any unwanted chemicals appear, neutralising and eradicating them, yet some will, without a doubt, get through.

Therefore, when it comes to skincare, organic verses normal high street, your skin is probably more than adequate at dealing with both. They are designed to be applied on your face and would have been tested and approved before production, so please don't worry unnecessarily about it. Organic is, of course, lovely and should you have the means, wonderful. When it comes to selecting your products, it is more about getting the right ingredients in those products to help your skin.

Note: I would like to briefly highlight household cleaning products. People get so wrapped up in considering their face products and what they put on their skin, yet spray all sorts around the house when cleaning. These products will indirectly come in contact with your face and hands. As these are not designed for topical application and are often a lot harsher, I would like to raise awareness of them and recommend looking for gentle cleaning products for your bathroom, living room and kitchen. For those with sensitive skin, you may be surprised at what a difference this makes to your skin.

Chapter 3:
Identifying Skin Type

Skin types once identified tend to remain the same throughout your life changing primarily only when you are younger, from a child into adolescence and when older; especially for a woman as your skin changes as a result of menopause. Although your skin may go through small bouts of unusual activity from time to time, perhaps dryness, spots, sensitivity. It's behaviour is normally triggered by external factors, being run down or unwell, or a reaction to a product and will resume back to its natural state once the body has rebalanced itself and/or treatment has been given.

Normal Skin

- Very few imperfections

- Calm skin (no known sensitivities)

- Barely visible pores

- Healthy radiant complexion

- Even skin tone

Oily

- Larger pores

- Often shiny appearance to the skin all over

- Prone to blackheads, whiteheads and spots

Combination

- A mixture where there are both dry/normal areas and oily areas, in various zones across the face.

- A t-zone is often quite common, where the nose, chin and forehead tend to produce more oils then the rest of the face, which tends to be normal or dry.

Dry

Please be aware having tightness does not necessarily mean you have a dry skin type, dehydration (lack of water) in the skin is different from dryness (lack of oil). Temporary dehydration can be easily treated with a good moisturiser and some hydration masks and your skin should resume back to its normal state. If the perceived dryness comes and goes you are not a dry skin type, you are another skin type, suffering from dehydration.

•Dry skin is lacking in oil

•Rougher texture to the skin

•Sometimes dry flakes or patches are visible

•Often feels tight after washing

•Red patches (sometimes dry areas can become irritated or inflamed)

•Almost invisible pores

•Premature fine lines may be more visible

Sensitive

A sensitive skin type is like this constantly; sensitivities do not come and go.

Note: If you have had a reaction to a product causing you sensitivity, whereby your skin then returns to normal, this makes you product sensitive (a reaction to an ingredient/s) not a sensitive skin type.

•Often prone to allergies

•Sensitive to external stimuli, often becoming red or blotchy

•Can feel tight after washing

•Thin epidermis

•Prone to dry flaky patches and broken capillaries

Essential Skin Care

Chapter 4:
Cleansing Effectively

The Difference between a Simple and a really Effective Cleanse

Every day our skin is subject to the environment, walking down the street our skin is covered with pollution, smoke, exhaust fumes and dust particles, so cleansing at the end of the day is essential.

Our skin is the largest organ of the body. On a daily basis, it works to excrete waste products from the body through our pores from head to toe. As we go about our day, sedimentary particles continuously land on our skin. In fact, next time you pass your window ledge or car on the way to work, feel free to swipe your finger across it. That beautiful layer of dirt is what your face is subjected to daily, through the environment.

Cleansing at the end of the day is truly essential. No one can truly achieve healthy glowing clear skin without cleansing on a daily basis.

For those who wear makeup and do not cleanse properly, this will only compound the situation. Allowing fine layers of makeup, mixed with pollution and dirt to accumulate, will no doubt contribute to blocked pores. Causing the build-up of oil from your sebaceous glands to become trapped leading to blackheads, whiteheads and pustules.

In fact, the best-case scenario you can hope for, for someone who doesn't cleanse properly, will be dullness and a lack of radiance to the skin.

The 'Splash'

A lot of ladies over the years have come to me concerned with the appearance and congestion of their skin and when I ask them 'how do you cleanse?' They say 'I splash with water'. This will not effectively cleanse the skin and has no ability to break down oils. As you know, oil and water don't mix. After re-educating them, I send them away with a gentle yet effective cleanser, 90% of all their problems stem from this one simple mistake.

Rule No.1# Cleanse the skin on a daily basis with cleanser. No questions.

Why cleanse both morning and evening?

Like I mentioned before your skin is a living organ and it will naturally produce sebum throughout the night, regardless of how effectively you have cleansed that evening. This is good; natural oils are beneficial to the skin, however gently cleansing in the morning will encourage the regulation of oil flow in the skin, and help pores to remain healthy and clear of excess debris and oils. Therefore, please do take the time to cleanse both morning and evening with a gentle cleanser.

Rule No. 2# Cleanse both AM and PM.

Make Up – The Golden Two-Part Rule

Make-up itself doesn't clog the pores.

Makeup has improved so much over the last decade. Formulations are now often created with skincare in mind. The majority are explicitly designed not to block pores. After all which company would want to create a product designed to give customers an outbreak of spots? Obviously, the formulations do vary from company to company, as a general rule look out for formulations that say they are non-comedogenic. These are products that are formulated not to cause blocked pores and work with your skin.

When I joined the skincare and cosmetic industry many years ago, I wore a full face of makeup as required by contract five days a week. While my skin was never truly bad, I did suffer from a few spots consistently on the go and made the assumption it was my foundation, which I blamed entirely for the state of my skin. I was cleansing once in the morning and once in the evening using a facial wash. Being a commuter, I was tired in the evening and felt that one cleanse was all I had the energy to muster. It wasn't until I was speaking to others in the industry, all who wore a full face of makeup daily and still had beautiful skin, that I realised the difference between their routine and mine, was one simple step, the 'double cleanse'.

From that time on I decided to adopt this approach in my evening skincare ritual and cleanse my skin thoroughly, the results were amazing. I still wear some of those foundations regularly to this day, yet without any issues. Who'd have thought an extra application and rinse taking 20 seconds would make such a difference to skin clarity.

Rule No.3# If you are wearing makeup double cleanse, the first cleanse will wash the makeup off; the second will cleanse the skin. It is a two-part rule.

If wearing makeup, don't make the mistake of believing one use of a cleanser will remove all products and pollution from the face, especially if wearing a long-lasting formulation. The first cleanse will wash the makeup off, the second will cleanse the skin.

Invest in the second Cleanse

The second cleanse is that investment time. It is the step that makes the difference, so if you're going to do it, I would recommend optimising results with the use of a facial cleansing aid, such as a facial sponge, flannel, cloth or cleansing device. But please cleanse and replace regularly. Therefore, please pick one that fits in with your lifestyle and maintenance routine. Do you prefer to throw things in the wash and recycle them, or throw them away and replace with a new item when they get grubby? If you are going to be massaging your face with whatever cleansing method you prefer, make sure you maintain hygiene standards.

A cloth/flannel should be used twice once in the morning and once in the evening, then hung up to dry in the interim. (A wet bundle in a ball will just promote bacterial growth). I would recommend holding a seven-day supply. This way you can continue your routine while some are in the wash without having to stop or extend the use of your last cloth.

A facial sponge should be rinsed after each use and left to air dry. I personally change mine the moment the brilliant white colour starts to fade. For me personally, this averages every three/four weeks.

If you're using a Sonic Brush, the recommendation is to replace the brush head every three months and to give it a good rinse weekly, allowing it to air dry after each use.

Yet again, I'm going to repeat myself here; you don't want to be using your sonic brush directly on makeup, vibrating and oscillating your make-up deep into to your pores. Cleanse the skin as you would normally, then use your cleansing brush on the final cleanse of the skin. This will also prevent staining your brush head, preserving it for longer, having the added benefit of saving you money as well.

What if I don't wear makeup- I am singularly cleaning my skin both morning and evening, should I still invest in cleansing aids?

Yes.

If you don't wear makeup and are singularly cleansing both morning and evening, I would still recommend investing, enhancing that 'one-off cleanse' so it achieves maximum results for you.

Rule No.4# Invest in your cleansing method of choice, apply daily and maintain and replace as required.

Cleansing- should always be gentle and never over strip the skin! There is no reason that cleansing has to be harsh. Cleansing should be effective, not stripping.

Recommended cleansers for different skin types

Cleansers for dry or sensitive skin

I would personally avoid any cleanser with sulphates in. The lathering agent sodium lauryl sulphate is the most common one used as a foaming agent in many cleansers, including shower gels, hand washes and hair shampoos. Sodium Lauryl Sulphate, in particular, is known to be very drying and may be a contributing factor to that tightness you feel after cleansing. There are many cleansers which cleanse the skin thoroughly avoiding sulphates that can produce a foam naturally or simply don't lather. For anyone suffering from dehydration or discomfort while cleansing, this may be a simple swap you can make to your routine, which is less drying on the skin.

Cleansers for oily or more combination skin

For you, I feel the risk is greater. I'm thinking in particular of those cleansers designed for spot prone skin, with claims of drawing out excessive oils. Beware of over stripping an oily/combination skin type, as this will cause your skin to produce more oil to compensate. Your body's natural defence is to rebalance the oils in the skin, creating harmony, for an oily skin, this means further production of oil, exacerbating the problem. It can also remove that equilibrium of healthy bacteria and natural oils needed for skin health and increase sensitivities. It is important to find a good effective cleanser that works for your skin that is still gentle and not over drying.

If suffering from blocked pores, spots or congestion, it may be worth looking out for a cleanser containing the ingredient salicylic acid. For more information on this ingredient, please see the chapter on exfoliators. Salicylic Acid is an exfoliator designed to help de-clog your inner pores. Used on a more consistent basis, this ingredient can really help prevent the build-up of blockages preventing clogged pores. However, although found in some cleansers it is more effective when on the skin for a prolonged period of time. A cleanser does not allow this to happen and I do not condone leaving cleansers on the skin for extended periods of time; as this has the potential to irritate the skin. Although this ingredient may help, I would personally recommend investing in other products containing salicylic acid; one that you are likely to leave on the skin for prolonged periods of time (such as a moisturiser or as an exfoliator which you can sweep over the skin with a cotton pad) and instead using a gentle cleanser, to effectively cleanse with thoroughly.

Oily skin with sensitivity or combination skin with sensitivity

In this case, please refer back to my original reference regarding sulphate free cleansers, as a gentle non-drying way to effectively cleanse the skin.

> *Rule No. 5# Consistently cleanse the skin with a gentle cleanser.*

Chapter 5:
The Mystery of a Toner

What is the benefit of using a toner, why should I use one?

I can't tell you how many countless times I've been asked this over the span of my career. Depending on the brand you use toners vary immensely. A good toner should be designed to rebalance the skin, providing a great line of defence between cleansing and moisturising, providing you pick the right one for your skin. Even the gentlest cleansers, including water (which may come as a shock to some), will alter the pH of the skin slightly, so this provides the perfect opportunity to give the skin what it needs, a balanced PH.

Rule No.6# Your toner should be pH balanced.

What should I look for in a good toner?

A good toner will be designed to balance the skin, leaving the skin at the correct pH. Normal healthy skin is slightly acidic with a pH of 5.5 this step is particularly important if the cleanser you are using is not pH friendly. A healthy pH will mean lipids and moisture will be balanced and your skin can effectively work at its best to block germs pollution and any toxins and bacteria.

It should ideally protect the skin with a combination of antioxidants, which will help prevent free radical damage (cell damage), aiding in the prevention of premature ageing.

Your toner should also preferably provide any extra active ingredients, depending on skin type to either hydrate, calm or purify the skin, allowing you to tailor the toner to your skin's needs.

Any toner chosen should not contain any ingredients which may cause damage to the skin with prolonged use. Alcohol denant is one of these.

Good VS Bad Alcohol

Not all alcohols are bad for the skin. Fatty alcohols are gentle and shouldn't irritate the skin; these include Cetyl, St Earyl, and Ceteryl. Small amounts are fine for any skin type, including dry skin and keep ingredients stable. So therefore I can't truly say to avoid all toners with alcohol.

However, the opposite is true of SD or Denatured alcohol. Another one to avoid is Isopropyl Alcohol but is less common in products now. Over time, these can weaken the skin, often causing dryness, redness and irritation in the process. I would strongly recommend avoiding any toners which contain these ingredients, especially if they are found anywhere within the top six ingredients in the ingredient list. In fact, I would go as far as to say avoid any products with these in, especially if you suffer from any sensitivity.

Rule No. 7# Avoid Denatured Alcohol, often seen as Alcohol Denant!! (SD/Isopropyl Alcohol)

Warning for those who are buying more astringent toners, take special care with the ingredients. Always remember to be gentle to your skin, after all the toner you choose will remain on your skin all day. You don't want it to unbalance the skin. If on application, you feel any stinging, heat, itchiness or redness avoid it, this is not the toner for you, throw it away! Your toner should leave your skin calm and refreshed.

Is a toner worth investing in?

There are a lot of people on the fence with this, whether to invest in a toner or not. I believe this is very much down to the stereotype of what a toner is and not really understanding what a toner should be. Remember you are buying a toner predominantly for protection and balance, the complete opposite of its perceived stereotype. Having a product which provides you with anti-oxidant protection and a balanced pH, is not to be underestimated.

According to Patricia Wexler M.D, a New York City dermatologist, interviewed for an article –'Key to great skin' by Karina Giglio,"if your skin becomes too alkaline, your skin becomes dry and sensitive and you may even get eczema." "while go the other way, although uncommon to become too acidic, the result is often breakouts, with red skin, inflamed and painful to touch." In my eyes, especially if you're not using pH balanced products, this can only be seen as a positive addition to any skincare routine.

Do toners shrink pore size?

No. Toners don't shrink pore size; however, toners can close pores.

Toners can't officially change the size of pores, but when looking at the visibility of pores, they can help tighten and close the pores, making them look visibly smaller. That is the keyword 'visibly'. Most toners focus on the claims of appearance. The 'appearance of pores are visibly reduced'.

For information on pores, please see the chapter on Skin Concerns - PORES.

"I have sensitive skin, so I tone with water"

Often people ask about splashing the face with water. Yes, just like warm water causes your pores to open a splash of cold water will close the pores, helping reduce the visibility to some extent, be it temporary. But unlike a toner, water doesn't contain any of the other benefits a good toner will provide, including antioxidant protection and the ability to balance the pH. Also, water (which is slightly more alkaline then our skin) if left to evaporate off the skin directly, can lead to dehydration of the surface skin cells.

Chapter 6:
What to Look for in a Moisturiser

Moisturisers are intended to hydrate the skin and treat dehydration. Face moisturisers work by holding onto water in the outermost layer of the skin.

The most beneficial time to moisturise is after a bath or shower, or after washing the face, as contact with hot or warm water will dehydrate the skin. I would also recommend bumping up the hydration if you have been out all day, particularly if you've been in the sun, as your skin is likely to be dehydrated from sun exposure.

Should oily skin types moisturise?

Yes!

Oily skin can still be dehydrated. If you have been in the sun all day, an oily skin can easily become dehydrated.

Dehydration leads to premature ageing and wrinkles. For those concerned with preventing this, even an oily skin will benefit from a light moisturiser. Look for a moisturiser designed to help combat dehydration. There are also some lovely oil-free ones on the market.

Dry skin type- what should I look out for in a good moisturiser?

For a dry skin type, I would recommend a moisturiser with a higher oil content. As dry skin, as you probably remember from the start of this book is caused by a lack of oil in the skin.

Dehydrated skin – Anyone with tightness?

For those with dehydrated skin, I would recommend looking at a moisturiser with Hyaluronic Acid. These great little molecules produced naturally in the skin will attract water, and retain it until needed, expanding in size as they hold onto the water. In fact, hyaluronic acid can hold onto up to 1000 times its weight in water. It is fantastic for hydration and plumping the skin, especially dehydration lines and brilliant for anyone suffering from dehydration or tightness in the skin. Suitable based on my own experience, and that of my customers, for those suffering from sensitive skin.

Rule No.8# Moisturise according to how your skin feels

When it comes to moisturising, always listen to your skin. Only you can tell if it needs a light or heavy cream, if it needs moisturising daily or twice daily. There is no set guideline; everyone's skin is different. But don't underestimate the benefit of hydration, for those who want radiant, glowing skin, ensure it is not dehydrated and moisturise regularly.

Rule No.9# The more hydrated your skin is, the more radiant it will look.

Chapter 7:
The Importance of Sunscreen

Sunscreen is designed to absorb or reflect some of the suns UV (Ultraviolet) radiation, helping to prevent these rays from reaching the skin. UV radiation is light from the sun in the form of wavelengths.

UVB a shorter wavelength is most commonly known for causing sunburn, skin damage and skin cancer*.

UVA the longer wavelength is known for causing skin damage and ageing as well as skin cancer.*

*www.skincancer.org

UVB and SPF Calculations

These days sunscreen commonly comes with a (Sun Protection Factor) SPF, this measures the sunscreens ability to prevent UVB damage to the skin. Measuring how long you can stay out in the sun before UVB rays start to burn your skin.

The rule of thumb is to be aware of how long you usually take to burn without SPF protection. You then multiply that time by the SPF factor chosen in your sunscreen to give you an indication of how long you can stay in the sun without burning.

So, in my case say my average burn time is 20 minutes and I want to wear a SPF 15 sunscreen:

SPF 15 x 20 mins =300 mins (5 hours)

SPF 15 x 10 mins =150 min (2hours 30mins)

However, please don't think wearing an SPF 50 will give you protection for the whole day, perspiration and other contributing factors will affect the longevity of protection and no sunscreen will block out all UVB rays. Even a SPF 50 only blocks out 98% or rays in full effect and an SPF 15 only 93% of UVB radiation.

The recommended reapplication of any sunscreen regardless of SPF is to reapply every two hours.

This is especially true if you are going swimming or heavily sweating, in which reapplication is recommended straight away. Companies are now no longer allowed to use phrases such as 'waterproof' or 'sweatproof', products can only be considered 'resistant'. Water resistant and sweat resistant products on average will provide you with only 40 mins up to 80mins of protection when under duress. They must then be re-applied.

UVA and Ageing

UVA is one of the main contributors to the development of wrinkles, loss of firmness and melanomas/skin cancer. You cannot feel it; it has no signal or sign, no redness or inflammation which you get when dealing with UVB rays. It is there always silently affecting your skin and, in my view, this makes UVA rays one of the most dangerous.

I once had a visitor to my counter who shared a story with me. She showed me a photo she got from YouTube. A truck driver went to work the same way every day, with the hot sun shining on one side of his face. By the time he had finished his deliveries, the sun had moved around, so the sun shone on that same side for his return journey. After years of doing this, one side as you can imagine had aged dramatically faster. His face was practically split down the middle; one side looked like the man was in his 70's, the other side like a man in his early 40's. Then, she let the bombshell drop. The driver said he always had had the windows up because he liked the air conditioning on. Just goes to show windows do not equal a barrier.

If you sit by a window UVA rays will penetrate, you are offered some protection from UVB rays as they are the wrong length to penetrate glass but not from UVA. Therefore, it is important to consider UVA also when deciding on a sunscreen, be it for your face or body.

Be aware, there are some sunscreens on the market that do not block UVA. A new legislation in the EU has outlined that UVA protection should now be at least one-third of the SPF. To help consumers a star rating system has now been introduced 1* (star) being the lowest UVA protection 5*(star) being the highest. Although not adopted everywhere yet it is becoming more common and does provide a useful awareness allowing you to consider both UVA protection and SPF when choosing a sunscreen.

However, as the star rating is not always found, please look at the ingredient list for UVA effectiveness. Make sure your sunscreen has at least one of the following:

Ecamsule, oxybenzone, avobenzone, titanium dioxide, zinc oxide or sulisobenzone.

As a guideline, both Titanium Dioxide and Zinc Oxide both give good UVA protection and have been around for years and are commonly found in most sunscreens (even those of a lower price bracket) and are gentle on sensitive skins. If comparing the two, Zinc Oxide is slightly superior as it covers a few more wavelengths, providing slightly greater protection.

Both for your own protection and to help prevent damage to your skin, use a broad-spectrum sunscreen with protection from both UVA and UVB.

Rule No.11# Use a broad-spectrum sunscreen with both UVA and UVB protection on a daily basis.

Even on a cloudy overcast day, 40% of UV radiation will still come through; therefore, the daily application of sunscreen is strongly recommended.

Note: Anyone over the age of 6 months should wear a SPF daily. Anyone under 6 months old should not wear sunscreen but should avoid sun exposure, as their skin is unable to process the chemicals found in sunscreen. They should, therefore, be covered and kept in the shade, out of direct sunlight at all times.

What's the difference between a physical sunscreen and a chemical sunscreen?

Sunscreen is one of two types either a 'physical sunscreen' that reflects light or a 'chemical sunscreen' that absorbs light preventing penetration. Both will effectively protect the skin from sun damage.

What factor SPF should I wear daily?

The choice is ultimately yours, but I certainly wouldn't wear anything lower than SPF 15 on a daily basis. While a SPF 30 or 50 is recommended if you are exposed to the sun for prolonged periods of time, there is a history of cancer in the family, you are fair skinned and prone to burning or you are concerned with the prevention and delay of ageing on the skin.

Also, be aware, some formulations are designed for everyday use while others are designed to be more resistant to heat, sweat and water. If you are out all day and in climates that promote sweating, or you are in going to be in contact with light showers or heavy rain, please make sure formulations selected are more water resistant and durable for protection.

Layering SPF

If I wear a SPF15 moisturiser and a foundation with SPF 15 what factor SPF do I have?

You would have a sun protection factor of 15 e.g. SPF 15.

SPFs can't be added together. The highest factor you apply is the highest protection you receive. The same is true if you apply regularly throughout the day. The SPF won't ever increase, but you will maintain that optimum level of protection.

Can I use sunscreen designed for adults on my children?

Babies over 6 months and children have sensitive skin, so it is best to avoid sunscreens designed for adults. Children's sunscreens are designed to be less irritating and will use ingredients like titanium dioxide and zinc oxide which are designed to reflect UV rays (physical sunscreen) unlike chemical sunscreens designed to absorb UV rays often found in adult sunscreens.

I have sensitive skin /rosacea, what would I benefit most from?

You may prefer formulations designed for children as these tend to be 'physical based' sunscreen. Physical based sunscreens are the recommended preference for those with sensitive skin. Look out for sunscreens with titanium dioxide or zinc oxide instead of chemical sunscreens. Avoid para-aminobenzoic acid (PABA), dioxybenzone, oxybenzone, or sulisobenzone commonly found in chemical sunscreens.

Will I get a vitamin D deficiency if I wear SPF regularly?

Although there has been some controversy regarding this, there is no known evidence that wearing SPF will lead to a vitamin D deficiency. Vitamin D helps the body absorb calcium and phosphate from our diet, which is important for healthy bones, teeth and muscles.

The recommended amount of sun exposure is 5-30 minutes twice a week, on either face, arms or legs. The amount of time needed will vary, influenced by factors such as cloud cover, the amount of skin exposed at any one time, and your skin colour. Those with darker skins (Asian, African, African-Caribbean), will need to spend more time in the sun, compared to someone with a lighter skin tone, to make the same amount of Vitamin D.

Just a quick reminder, Vitamin D is produced through exposure to UVB rays. If you are sitting by a window enjoying the sun this won't be contributing to making Vitamin D, as UVB rays can't penetrate glass, unlike UVA rays; you will need to venture outside and brave the fresh air. Vitamin D can also be obtained through supplements and a select number of foods, including egg yolks, oily fish (such as salmon, sardines & mackerel) and red meat and fortified spreads. Throughout winter this can be a good way to top up your vitamin D levels. For an average person getting the recommended amount of Vitamin D is easily achievable, especially during the summer months, and during winter your body is likely to use foods to supplement the amount of Vitamin D created when the sunlight levels are lower. For those concerned this provides an alternative way to top up your Vitamin D levels, through a healthy and natural diet, without putting yourself at risk of overexposure to UV rays, allowing you to wear sun protection without concern.

For those who are bed-bound, an extra focus on diet and/or supplements will be particularly important, to ensure good vitamin D levels.

It's cloudy outside, should I bother with sunscreen?

Yes. 40% of UV radiation still reaches the earth on a cloudy day. Just because it's cloudy doesn't mean you stop wearing sunscreen. You may spend all day outside without sun protection; done regularly this can lead to serious skin damage. So always wear a broad-spectrum UVA/UVB sunscreen.

Chapter 8:
Serum

An exciting new market has emerged over the last decade, which has completely taken the skincare industry by storm, the emergence of the super serum. Serums are designed to be made up of concentrated ingredients targeting specific results, which have the ability to travel deeper into the skin; promising results more quickly than a moisturiser.

They often come with separate or multiple benefits including improved hydration, anti-ageing results focusing on reducing the appearance of lines and wrinkles and improving the firmness and elasticity of the skin. Some look at enhancing the radiance of the skin, while some are designed to minimise the appearance of pores and mattify the skin. While others help even out your skin tone and pigmentation, the list goes on...They are designed to be applied under your moisturiser to bump up results. With serums being either oil or water-based, you can select the right type of serum to complement your skin type.

Can I use a serum as an alternative moisturiser?

Through personal experimentation, the majority of serums will provide hydration benefits to the skin and although this might sound rather blasphemous, for those with a combination or oily skin, if you're struggling to find the right moisturiser, you could always use the serum as an alternative. As they are normally designed to be applied after toning and before moisturising, they are designed to feel light on the skin and are absorbed well. Just look for a water-based serum specifically. This could also be an alternative for someone with oily or more combination skin. Rebellious I know, but I promise I won't tell anyone of your secret.

While for those with dryer skin type I would not recommend this as an alternative to a moisturiser, a moisturiser will provide a higher level of comfort to the skin. Instead, I would recommend adding the serum underneath your moisturiser as an added boost. Although you can use any of your choice, you may find an oil-based serum gives you more benefits. For those with normal or combination skin, you have the option to experiment.

If you do decide to use a serum only, don't forget to add a SPF on top.

Serums are usually more expensive than moisturisers because of the increased concentration of ingredients, but if you do want to achieve targeted results, this is one of the best ways you can go about it. One pump a day helps keep those annoyances away!

Rule No.12# Have a concern? Look for a serum on the market designed to target it, serums provide more concentrated and focused results, in a faster time frame.

Chapter 9: Exfoliators

The Difference between Good and Superb Skin!

Exfoliation is one of the most, and I'll repeat this, THE most important contributions to glowing skin, texture and appearance. A large power busting deterrent in keeping pores clear and congestion at bay, with the added benefit of improving skin texture and appearance, and making any makeup application appear smoother.

Exfoliation can be done in so many different ways, both manually with a traditional product such as a scrub, or chemically via application of fruit acids.

Manual Exfoliation

Scrubs

When it comes to manual exfoliation, most people think of traditional scrubs. Scrubs contain beads or small fragments of natural ingredients, biodegradable by choice if you are conscious of the environment. These are massaged onto clean damp skin, effectively exfoliating away dead skin cells.

Scrubs can be effectively used after cleansing twice a week or if suffering from dry areas, visible flakes or dry patches of skin to the touch, every third day. Using light gentle pressure, this is a lovely way to gently exfoliate the skin.

Daily face scrubs in the guise of cleansers

I would personally avoid these. Manually buffing your skin with particles on a daily basis, no matter how gentle they claim to be, can tend to over stimulate the skin and cause sensitivity. Instead look for other ways to gently remove dead skin cells on a daily basis, without particles or beads.

Daily Buffing

Gentle Daily buffing is maintenance and should be carried out alongside any 'proper' or 'deeper' exfoliation. I say this as daily buffing should leave your skin in a calm state. It provides an improved cleansing habit which ever so slightly ups your daily exfoliation, but through consistency helps prevent blocked pores, cleanses more efficiently and improves the radiance of the skin. Your personal choice of method, whether you use a cloth, flannel, sponge or even a sonic brush can be selected by yourself.

My Personal Favourite- soft facial sponge

I invested in the masses of products to help cleanse and buff my skin daily and I have to say my firm favourite is a soft facial Sponge. It costs me about £4 and I replace it monthly, very simple, gentle, yet effective.

I use this to massage my cleanser into my skin morning and evening to effectively cleanse my skin, I then integrate other methods of exfoliating throughout the week to target the maintenance of my pores.

Like I said, I've dabbled and stopped using it for a couple of years, while I tried other gentle ways of buffing the skin daily. Having gone back to it again and seen the difference in my skin, I feel I now couldn't be without it. Everyone is different, find your preferred method.

Rule No.13# Learn exfoliation is not about intensity it's about gentle consistency.

Very gently buff the skin every day when cleansing, to provide gentle exfoliation consistently; whether this is once a day or twice a day is completely up to you, as always listen to your skin.

Glycolic Acid (AHA) – Super Smoother

Glycolic acid is a water-soluble acid know as an AHA (alpha hydroxy acid), commonly found in various fruits and milk. It is great for smoothing the skin, improving skin texture and appearance.

If you don't like manual exfoliation in the form of scrubs or other methods, or you aren't seeing the results, or you simply want a really effective exfoliator with minimal effort, then I would recommend the use of an AHA like Glycolic Acid.

The use of a product containing this ingredient can be a great way to speed up the process of improving surface texture and the appearance of the skin. Achieving a more even skin tone, as you resurface the face gently over time. With use it encourages the top layer of dead skin cells to shed more quickly, leaving you with a brighter, more even skin surface.

•It is beneficial for those with dry skin; suffering from flakes or dry patches.

•As well as for those who want to speed up cell turnover, to help remove visible marks from the skin. (This would apply to red marks or decolourisation left over from an occasional spot, often in the form of a pink mark, that would on average normally take two or three months to fade naturally. Glycolic Acid can really speed up the turnaround of this. (Please note this will not have the same effect on pigmentation/ dark spots/age spots).

•Glycolic Acid is also particularly good for helping with fine lines and wrinkles, reducing visibility over time.

Glycolic Avid comes in various concentrations, starting at around 5-10% up to higher concentrations. However, the FDA (www.fda.gov) does state that *"concentrations above 10% for fair skins may be too much, causing skin irritation".

Under no circumstance would I recommend using any Glycolic Acid with a concentration above 10%, unless applied by a professional. A higher concentration will need a neutraliser, and your skin's reaction and results can vary with higher concentrations.

The pH of the product will also determine the strength of the product, so a 10% concentration in one product may differ from a 10% concentration from another. The higher the pH of the product the less effective it will be.

As a guideline, AHAs like glycolic acid work best at concentrations of 5-10% within a pH of 3-4. My recommendation is to start with a low percentage say 5%

and see how you go. Always seek professional advice if in doubt.

A 5% concentration is widely considered a gentle concentration for the skin. Unfortunately I can give you no guideline as to application, as depending on the concentration and individual product, the time frame would differ. Some products allow you to wear it all throughout the night as a treatment, others for only a short space of time; sometimes only minutes. Similarly, the frequency of use will vary. Some will allow weekly treatments, others fortnightly, some more frequent, some even daily.

Glycolic Acid is well recognised and wildly available as an exfoliator and can be found in your local cosmetic/beauty hall with ease. It is popular also because when maintained, you tend to see results quite quickly, in comparison to say more traditional methods such as facial scrubs. Both of which target the surface layer of the skin.

Other known AHA's although less widely used include lactic acid, citric acid, tartaric acid, and malic acid.

Best Exfoliator for Black Heads and Pores
BHA- Salicylic Acid

My favourite, this exfoliator works on the inside of the pores rather than on the surface layer of the skin.

BHA'S such as Salicylic Acid are oil soluble. This allows them to penetrate the oils in the pores and exfoliate skin cells found inside the pores follicle, which has the tendency to clog. BHA's are really good at exfoliating the inner pores; therefore, absolutely great for helping to eliminate blackheads and blemishes.

Salicylic Acid comes in concentrations of 1%-2% found within products, most effective within a pH of 3-4. As salicylic acid is related to aspirin (both are salicylates), it can have an anti-inflammatory effect on the skin, reducing redness and swelling. In my experience my skin loves this ingredient, it is really good at preventing congestion and works wonders on my pores, but it can cause a hint of pinkness to my skin depending on which brand of product I decide to use. Others with less sensitive skin may find they don't suffer from this, so do have a play as to which product and formulation work best for you and in what concentrations. Products with1% or 2% Salicylic Acid are available in many forms, lotions, cream, gels, washes, or as a stand-alone exfoliator in its own right. Whether you use this daily, or every two or three days (as I do now for continuous maintenance, to help keep my pores clear), is completely up to you.

Be aware some products tend to add alcohol denant in with salicylic acid, with the assumption of large pores = oily skin and would benefit from a strong astringent. You know better and should avoid these products. Gentle but effective is always the best way to go.

Would you get quicker results from Scrubs or AHA's /BHA'S?

AHA'S and BHA's will provide more effective results because they work via a chemical process, they have a better ability to penetrate the top layers of the skin, to achieve results then a scrub would.

Therefore, for those with problematic skin and a blemished skin complexion, a combination of both inner pore exfoliation from salicylic and a glycolic peel or product for surface exfoliation can be effective. However only ever use one exfoliator at any one time and as always, of course, listen to your skin and adopt a routine that suits your skin.

Don't forget..

Always apply sun cream if using these exfoliators especially for a week afterwards, as your skin will be more sensitive to sunlight.

Can you over exfoliate?

Yes and no, yes regarding sensitivity but no in regards to your cells.

Yes, if you over exfoliate you will find your skin becomes irritated and inflamed. Reduce the frequency of exfoliation and/or the percentage of exfoliate used. Always listen to your skin. Find the right balance for you.

But No, you can't over exfoliate in the sense, you won't ever run out of skin cells. The purpose of exfoliation is to remove dead skin cells from the surface of the skin; this increases the production of new healthy skin cells to be formed. Increasing the rate at which your skin cells are shed and replaced or as we like to say in the business increasing the cell turnover.

Put simply the Basal Layer of the skin contains two types of cells, one which has a certain lifespan for reproduction referred to as the 'Hayflick limit', should you wish to look it up. The Hayflick limit basically refers to the fact that all healthy skin cells, can on average replicate only around 40-60 times only. This only applies to skin cells that are fully differentiated (cells with a purpose in their final state...you are to become a skin cell...) The other cells, called stem cells, have no reproduction limit and are the exception to the Hayflick limit. The stem cell which is undifferentiated, as of yet has no purpose, can turn into any cell that is required, including the new healthy skin cells we desire and can replicate as much as it wishes. So, you will always have skin cells available. These stem cells replicate as often as required throughout your whole life. So, feel free to exfoliate as often as you wish and enjoy the benefits. Like I mentioned before, find your individual perfect amount.

Rule No.14# supplement your daily buffing routine twice week with a deeper exfoliation.*

Note: BHAS' like Salicylic can be used more frequently, however sensitive skin types, or those suffering from rosacea; simply maintain daily buffing instead and do not supplement.

Chapter 10:
Masks

Masks are designed to treat the skin on a deeper level; they come in various formats such as:

•Hydration Masks, to rehydrate and soften the skin.

•Clay masks, designed to draw out excess oils and impurities in the skin.

•Brightening masks, to improve the radiance and glow the skin, often mixed with exfoliators or other active ingredients to help brighten the skin.

The great thing about masks is that nowadays there are so many available. There is one to suit every time frame, no longer is the excuse, 'I don't have time to do a mask', able to be used with sincerity'. Most masks take 10-15 minutes, some masks can be slept in, and others deliver results in anything from 30 seconds to 5 minutes. If you're concerned with fitting it into your lifestyle, have a look around, there are lots of options out there.

My favourite time to do a mask is when making a cup of tea in the morning, after washing my face. I like to make a cup of tea wearing the mask, by the time I have drunk my tea, it's time to remove the mask. For those of you, who think you don't have time, think outside of the box. A mask takes 30 seconds to apply and 30 seconds to rise off. You can do whatever you like for the rest of the time. Get something done or relax; the choice is yours.

Masks are so beneficial to the skin, think of it as doctors' orders. When your skin is playing up, this is when you should analyse what it needs and apply the appropriate mask. Providing your skin with the treatment it needs to get better.

Facial Mask Mapping

There is no rule you have to apply one mask all over. Yes, if your skin needs that particular benefit to apply it all over. However, if you're skin type is a combination like mine and some bits need hydration and other areas need oil absorption, zone of your face and apply your masks to different areas, without overlapping and have fun with it. I love a bit of facial mask mapping. Why stop at two? I might want an anti-ageing mask on my neck and forehead as well!

Not only will you provide the right needs for all the areas, but you also save time too! Bonus.

Listen to your skin on the day, identify and play. You'll get far better results.

How many times a week should you apply a mask?

As a guide, I would recommend applying a mask twice a week, once as a bare minimum, if using a manual exfoliator such as facial scrub etc... Apply the mask/s after rinsing off the scrub for maximum benefits. Exfoliating first will allow better penetration of the mask.

Chapter 11:
Home Facials-Amplify your Results

Key Step by Step Guide to carrying out your own Luxury Facial at Home

1) Double cleanse the skin thoroughly.

2) Use a facial scrub to eliminate dead skin cells, (do not use any other exfoliators AHA's or BHA's on the same day).

3) Steam the skin. Fill a heat proof bowl with boiling water; allow it to cool for 1-2 mins. Apply 2-3 drops of essential oils into the water, then sit with your head over the bowel and a towel draping over your head, trapping the steam. Please ensure during this time your eyes are closed, to prevent the essential oils irritating the eyes. Sit and inhale the steam for the relevant time, please see guideline below as to which essential oils would be most beneficial to you. This should be a comfortable and enjoyable procedure, if you find the steam is too hot, please move your face further away from the bowel to allow more air flow.

Steaming opens up the pores and softens the skin, encouraging the glands to produce more oils which eliminate waste. It improves circulation to the skin, aiding the flow of nutrients and carrying away waste. As well as softening oily deposits in follicles aiding comedone extraction.

The use of essential oils:

2-3 drops added into the water will provide an extra treatment for the skin.

•Tea tree- Beneficial if you have spots/congestion.

•Rosemary- Great for oily skin.

•Lavender- Suitable for all bar the most sensitive. Relaxing but also antibacterial and a decongestant.

•Jasmine- Great for dry skin.

•Geranium-Great normal skin, but a lovely alternative for all, great for brightening your mood.

•Eucalyptus- Wonderful if you have sinus congestion or dark circles.

How long to Steam for?

•Sensitive skin/ pregnant or nursing, steam the skin for 3-5 mins (Do not use essential oils.)

•Dry/more mature skin steam for 5 mins

•Normal or Combination steam for 5-10 mins

•Oily skin steam for 10 minutes.

4) Relax

5) Extraction

Once the skin is soft, it is now time for extraction should you have the need. Wrap some tissue around one finger on each hand leaving some excess tissue sticking up over the edge of the finger, fold the excess tissue over the top of the nail and down over the inside of the finger, then gently give the relevant area or pore a small squeeze. The tissue will stop your fingernail cutting into the skin, we don't want to scar the skin with your nail, neither do we want to traumatise the area. If the comedone, blackhead or whitehead, does not come out with one squeeze, it may not be ready. In which case leave it.

That's it resist! Do not go over the same area twice. Remember, this is a gentle aid to help, no extremism.

Otherwise, you have the potential to do more harm than good, remember we don't want to damage the pores.

Replace the tissue on each finger after each extraction, as you continue moving to different areas of the face.

6) Once any extractions have been done, sweep over with toner.

7) Then apply masks. Multi-map different masks onto different zones or apply all over face, avoiding eye area.

8) After applying your mask, use this time to RELAX. Relaxing and destressing are good for your skin also! Otherwise multi-task if you must, just because you have a mask on doesn't mean you can't do the washing up if you have to. However, in such a hectic world, it's nice to designate a bit of me time. 10-15 mins later depending on the mask instruction rinse or wipe off.

9) Tone- re-sweep the whole face to rebalance the pH.

10) Apply eye cream around the orbital bone (eye bone socket), using a sweeping movement starting outwards below the eye, sweep inwards towards the bridge of the nose and up over the eyebrows, sweeping outwards towards the temples.

11) Take the time to really massage the skin, applying any oils or serums to the face, (avoiding the eye area). Pick one relevant to your skin needs.

12) Moisturise. Allow 3-5 minutes for facial massage to help with circulation and blood flow. Close your eyes and enjoy the feeling of massaging the skin.

13) Lastly, take a minute, shut your eyes and do some slow controlled breathing.

How often should I do my own facial?

In an ideal world I would say twice a week, but as a golden rule at least once a week. As always listen to your skin. Its needs will vary from day to day.

Rule no.15# Aim to pamper yourself with a facial once a week. Really enjoy the experience.

Skin Conditions/Concerns

Most common Skin Concerns Start with Inflammation

Chapter 12: Whiteheads, Blackheads and Acne

What causes spots?

Each hair follicle grows from an oil gland and secretes sebum; they live within what is commonly known as a pore. When things are working as they should, the oil will easily leave the pore and provide moisture for the skin. The problems arise when the pore gets plugged with sebum and dead skin cells, providing an ideal environment for bacteria to grow, leading to the formation of a spot!

When you have too many dead skin cells on the surface of the skin and inside the pore and your skin cells are not being shred properly, the combination of any excess oil will mean the pore will become blocked. This lovely mixture will solidify as a white substance.

•If the surface of the pore is covered by skin you have a white head.

*Milia is a form of white head; this is when there is a hard-white bump with no puss, swelling or redness.

•If the pore is open with no skin covering the surface, the top section of gunk will be exposed to air. Oxidation will then take place, which is what causes this lovely mixture to turn black and you have a black-head!

•Black-heads and whiteheads become spots when Propionibacterium acnes (P. Acnes) a type of bacteria starts to grow. A blocked pore full of sebum and dead skin cells is the perfect environment for this type of bacteria to thrive in. With this constant supply of sebum, it can reproduce, which is what causes irritation, inflammation and eventually ruptures the oil gland. The bacteria, oil and dead skin cells are let loose in the surrounding skin tissue. The body's immune system will respond by causing swelling, which is why spots are red and often swollen and inflamed. They can also be called or referred to as papules and pustules.

Acne affects 95% of the population at some point in their lives in various forms; from mild to severe.

The main triggers for spot creation include:

1) Overproduction of oil by sebaceous (oil) glands.

2) Changes in hormones. In particular, the overproduction of male hormones called androgens, which control oil production.

3) Dead skin cells on the surface of the skin (not enough shedding) and the inner pore (excessive shedding).

4) Build-up of bacteria.

5) Irritation.

Hormones are the biggest contributor to increased oil production

Although hormones can't create blemishes on their own, combine hormones with something going wrong, such as the oil flow in the inner pore being slowed or trapped, or perhaps you are not effectively exfoliating or cleansing properly, and you have a much larger chance of blemishes occurring.

Hormones are affected by:

•Pregnancy

•Birth control pills

•Menstrual cycle

•Stress

•Corticosteroids

•Foods- Although there is no conclusive official evidence on the subject yet, concerns preside over hormones added/found in chicken, beef and milk.

Overview- How to treat Blemishes

To treat blemishes and spots, you need to look at:

1) Reducing oil production

2) Reducing the amount of dead skin on the surface of the skin and in the inner pore

3) Killing any residing bacteria if present (P. acnes). This can be done using either topical and/or oral methods.

So how do you kill P. Acnes bacteria?

One of the most common products available on the market is Benzol Peroxide. When applied to the skin Benzoyl Peroxide releases oxygen in a free radical format on application to the skin. For those of you unaware P. acnes bacteria are not able to live in an oxygen rich environment. The oxygen produced by Benzol Peroxide 'burns', or irritates, the membrane of the bacteria cell. With the bacteria now diverting its energy into maintaining its outer membrane, it is more susceptible to the attack of our immune system. On average 98% of bacteria will die within 48 hours of application not having replicated, thus preventing more bacteria from being produced.

Benzoyl Peroxide is proven to be very effective on mild to moderate acne, but it can have side effects: redness, tingling, burning, itching and dryness, especially if using higher concentrations.

If you want to get rid of acne, but want to reduce the side effects of using this product then you should start with a 2.5% over-the-counter product, available from your local pharmacy. Or up to a 5.5% microsphere, time release benzoyl peroxide (BP) product (more likely available from your doctor), should your skin be OK with 2.5 % BP product. Solubilized microsphere benzoyl peroxide (newer on the market) not only kills bacteria in spots, but it also helps exfoliate dead skin cells, assisting pores to drain and is considered gentler on the skin as it releases small amounts slowly over time rather than in one big hit. A newer development considered *'more effective and kinder to the skin'.*www.facingacne.com

Awareness: Although you can get 10% Benzol Peroxide over the counter, this would not be suitable for application all over the face, rather used for direct application to individual spots, a low concentration would be best for treating the entire face. My younger sister made the mistake of this when she was a teenager and bought the 10% by accident and smeared it all over her face. Her skin was red raw.

According to clinical studies *'lower concentrations are just as effective as high concentration and cause less irritation'. *www.acne.com

If you have rosacea, I would avoid benzoyl peroxide, as inflammation and irritation is a trigger for the creation of spots. Such a sensitive skin may react in a more extreme way, which has the potential to trigger the creation of new small spots.

Also, if you have Asian skin, or darker skin, failure to use sun protection when you use benzoyl peroxide may result in brown discolouration of the skin, so either avoid and seek other treatments or remember to use a SPF daily.

For anyone using Benzoyl Peroxide, be aware of your bed sheets. It does have the potential to fade and discolour coloured fabrics. Cotton is particularly vulnerable. Opt for white sheets, linen's, pillowcases and pyjamas instead, as they can't be bleached by Benzoyl Peroxide. Also remember to wash your hands thoroughly after applying, so as not to affect your hand towels. Yet again the 'white rule' would be best adapted to hand towels temporarily while using.

Alternative light therapy

For those with sensitive skin or for those who do not wish to apply topical products on the skin, light therapy may provide an alternative for you.

How Light Therapy Works:

Dermatologists have used light therapy for over a decade. Although trials have been done on small groups of people, with very promising results, as of yet, there has not been a large long-term study.

LED lights work by gently penetrating the skin at various depths to stimulate the skin's physiology. Blue light targets acne, killing bacteria while red light reduces acne inflammation. Designed to treat mild to moderate acne.

You can purchase handheld devices, which require you to hold the device directly on an area or several areas of your face. More recently, light masks have been produced which allows the user to wear a light mask covering their whole face.

If you have more than the occasional few spots, a mask may be better as it would require less time to apply to each area of concern before moving on to the next, as it would cover a much larger surface area. If time wasn't a factor or your spots and blemishes are few, devices designed for smaller areas are much cheaper. The recommended length of time varies depending on the device, usually anywhere from 3-4 mins on singular spots, to fifteen minutes and half hour treatments on larger areas.

With a daily or twice daily treatment, results range from a few days for treatment of an individual spot to four to twelve weeks for visible results on moderate acne.

Blue light study:

Some promising studies have reported that physician-administered blue light therapy of 30 people showed results of *57% to 73% reduction in acne after 5 weeks, with effects lasting in the weeks following treatment. With 77% showing improvement in 5 weeks and 40% showing marked improvement or clearance of the acne.

*www.acne.org

Another study on 23 people having treatment twice a week for 15 mins over the course of four weeks showed *80% responded to treatment, showing a 59-67% reduction of inflammatory acne lesions. For more information on statistics, please see www.acne.org.

Red light:

Researcher performed a study on 30 people to investigate the effectiveness of physician-administered red-light therapy as a stand-alone treatment. The study reported that *'red light therapy reduced non-inflammatory acne (whiteheads and blackheads) by 59% and inflammatory acne (papules and pustules) by 66%'.Reducing the number of acne spots but not removing them completely. After discontinuation of red light therapy acne resumed, highlighting continuous treatment would be needed to sustain results.'*www.acne.org

Best results were found with a mixture of blue and red light; results show a reduction in inflammatory lesions by 76-83%. Although the improvements were not significantly greater than the results using blue light alone, it would appear that combining both blue and red light gave better results. A lot of the devices available to buy now combine both blue and red light.

I have to say I own one of these devices, a small design intended to treat a small spot or two at a time. I have had great success with it. For someone with sensitive skin, this has proven to be a gentle and effective treatment when needed, without sensitising my skin.

Drying up spots...that doesn't make sense!

Drying up the skin is just depleting skin cells of water. This has no positive effect, as spots are worsened by oil production not excess water. So, please don't suddenly cut out your moisturiser if you see spots, or use very drying products on your skin in a desperate attempt to combat the situation. Dehydrating the skin of water will only leave the skin tight, dry and sensitive and less likely to heal, you want to be focused on ways to reduce oil production. One of the best and easiest ways I know to absorb excess oils is the use of a clay-based mask, to gently absorb excess oils. Used frequently this can be really effective and simple treatment to combat excess oils, without dehydrating the skin.

On the spot treatment

In my experience when people see spots, they panic and suddenly go out and buy a spot treatment designed to be applied topically to that area. Normally containing a higher concentration of exfoliator, or some kind of antibacterial property, commonly salicylic acid, witch hazel or tea tree… Ever done that?

While this may provide short-term relief, you should be aware a spot doesn't appear out of nowhere formed in minutes. It, in fact, takes around three weeks to develop. Therefore, you may be treating one now but it is highly likely, there are others in process. I strongly believe it would be better and far more prudent to add an exfoliator regularly into your routine to tackle spots not yet visible in prevention, rather than last-minute rescue attempts. 'Prevention is better than cure!'

Hang on I'm sure I've heard that somewhere before?...

Incorporate a consistent routine:

•Exfoliate regularly - preventing blocked pores.

•Disinfect or apply a product designed to kill bacteria if suffering from spots.

•Absorb excess oil regularly- clay-based masks are great for this.

•Care for skin, gently, effectively and consistently. Consistency is the key.

Hints and tips on helping to prevent self-sabotage

There are small things you can do to help stop the spread of bacteria and help you in your fight against spots:

•Hold your phone to your ear not your face, how many times have you smearily touched that screen and then press it to your cheek? Hmmm worth considering.

•Regularly clean your phone with screen wipes. How often do you do that?? Have you ever done that???

•Change your face towel once a week and ensure it is not damp and harbouring bacteria. Remember to hang it up to dry in between uses.

•If someone in your family also has acne, avoid sharing face cloths or towels.

•Don't touch your face or pick and squeeze spots or blackheads constantly. Extraction is beneficial when your fingers are clean, your skin has been prepared and it's done properly. However, even then it should be done in moderation. However, dirty fingernails will aggravate and damage the skin and spread bacteria to other parts of the face, compounding the problem, resist! No touching.

•Hair products (Shout out for guys in particular here). How often do you adjust your hair throughout the day, get your styling waxes and gels on your hands and then touch your face? Products like these leave a lovely residue which you don't want anywhere near your face! Try not to play with your hair throughout the day and if you catch yourself adjusting your hair in the mirror, wash your hands afterwards.

•Stress. When you're stressed your body produces cortisol, which tells glands in your skin to make more oil, a large contributor to the formation of blemishes. Take time every day, even if its' just for a few minutes to try and reach a state of calm. Long-term find activities that relax you and make them a priority. Exercise can also be a good stress reliever, whether it's walking or doing a class. Take the time to look after yourself inwardly a well as outwardly.

•Avoid eating an inflammatory diet, although this diet is not officially recognised, it's widely accepted that inflammation is at the heart of acne, therefore eating anti-inflammatory foods can only help your cause. Try eating a selection of leafy greens and vegetables and fruits high in antioxidants. Leafy greens like: spinach, kale and chard are great antioxidants and have great anti-inflammatory properties. Other great vegetables include broccoli, cauliflower and Brussel sprouts. Blueberries and pineapple are also great anti-inflammatories.

Chapter 13:
Pores

Enlarged pores are caused by debris inside the pores which has caused them to stretch, making them larger than they would normally be. If pores are left in this state for too long, you run the risk that the cellular structure of the pore becomes damaged and the pores remain in this state permanently. This is why it's so important you cleanse effectively and exfoliate regularly if you dream of small invisible pores. However, should your pores have become permanently damaged (I know there is one on my face which is permanently damaged and enlarged), there is only so much a good cleansing and exfoliating routine will do. Although you will see results, you have to accept they may never be the same as they once were. The trick is not to let them get to that point in the first place.

Chapter 14: Dark Circles

A lot of people suffer from dark circles under the eyes. Although you can take steps to cover dark circles with makeup, it's worth knowing a bit more about what forms dark circles in the first place and how to help prevent them.

Dark circles are predominantly the result of being able to see your blood vessels under the skin. It is not caused by tiredness or staying up too late. The skin around your eye area averages 0.5mm, making it 75% thinner than anywhere else, so when factors influence the dilation of blood vessels, they show up as dark circles.

People more inclined to suffer the effects of dark circles include:

•Those who genetically have thinner than the usual skin around this area, so constantly suffer from dark circles as a result.

•Those who are more elderly. As you age your skin is less able to regenerate, you have less collagen and elasticity in the skin and your skin becomes thinner increasing the visibility of blood vessels beneath.

•Those disposed to hyper-pigmentation, where more melanin is produced under the eye area making it look darker (melanin is what contributes to our tan); in most cases, this is more common in those with darker skin.

•Nasal congestion, this is probably one of the most common triggers. Whether that is a result of allergies (hay fever) or illness (cold/ flu), this causes the blood vessels around your eye area, which normally help with drainage to dilate, making them more visible and causing the eye area to darken.

•Medication, some prescriptions can lead to the dilation of the blood vessels around the eyes. For example, if you are suffering from the liver disease the medication you would be taking would certainly mean you are more prone to dark circles.

•Scratching or rubbing your eyes excessively, often those with allergies will inadvertently damage blood vessels around this area when suffering from hay fever.

•Anaemia (Iron deficiency) is one of the most common causes of inexplicable dark circles in many cases. Low iron levels result in poor oxygenation in body tissues, due to the low supply of oxygenated blood. This can be treated by making simple changes in your diet. If you suffer from low iron levels, try to consume a balanced diet, rich in green leafy vegetable (avoiding spinach), soybeans, lentils (including other forms of beans) such as chickpeas and kidney beans, to keep your body healthy and your iron level up. Red meat like beef and liver as well as mussels and oysters are excellent for iron levels also.

What Steps can I take to Reduce Dark Circles?

If you are not genetically pre-disposed to dark circles, there are various measures you can adopt to reduce dark circles around the eyes:

•Prevent dehydration by increasing the amount of water you consume. If you are suffering from nasal congestion, a higher intake of fluid will help with the drainage of mucus around the eye area.

•Cut down on things that increase dehydration, like alcohol, caffeine and sugar. Blood vessels constrict when dehydrated, this puts more pressure on them and can inadvertently lead to ruptures.

•Try to avoid rubbing the eye area if suffering from allergies and take special care when removing eye makeup, as over rubbing can cause damage to the blood vessels.

•Protect the eye area from the sun. Sun damage contributes to the weakening and thinning of the skin. This can make dark circles more prominent as the blood vessels are more visible. Wearing an SPF around the eye area, as well as sunglasses, will help to protect them from sun damage when out in the sun.

•Increase your intake of vitamin C which is known to strengthen blood vessels. This will also help to slow down ageing, which as mentioned before, contributes to the thinning of the skin around the eye area. Vitamin C is great at providing antioxidant protection from free radical damage. Vitamin C can be found in citrus fruit, as well as fruit such as red currants, blackberries, strawberries, raspberries and kiwis.

•Cut down or stop smoking. The increase in carbon dioxide lowers the oxygen contained within your blood, and de-oxygenated blood will show up as having more of a blue tinge.

•For those in need of a quick short temporary fix, a cold compress around the eye area can help shrink capillaries, so darkness is temporarily less apparent.

Chapter 15:
Eye Puffiness

Puffy bags below your eyes are almost always caused by fluid build-up, either due to illness, allergies or excessive salt consumption, which can result in the body retaining more fluid than usual. This can place increased pressure on the skin and blood vessels around your eyes, forcing blood vessels closer to the surface of the skin, making dark circles and puffiness more apparent.

Eye Drainage Massage for Puffiness

When next applying your eye cream of choice, I would recommend sweeping movements in the form of facial massage.

From the outside under eye area just below your temples, use your middle fingers to sweep inward towards the bridge of the nose following your orbital socket. Go up over the bridge of the nose, then circle back just under your eyebrows towards your temples forming a circle. Repeat six times. Do this a further six times, but this time repeat the movement using three fingers to sweep across the forehead (instead of under the brows), draining from the centre of the forehead to the temples, for increased drainage. Remember to extend out all the way to the temple, pause for a second and do a small clockwise rotation, then continue the movement for optimum drainage and relaxation. Pressure should be comfortable and smooth.

Repeated daily this can help reduce the appearance of fluid retention and aid drainage under the eye area.

Chapter 16: Eczema

Eczema is a continuous inflammation at a low level.

There are different types of eczema, the most common being atopic eczema (atopic dermatitis), 'atopic' means sensitivity to allergens. Eczema is commonly recognised when skin is itchy, dry, red and cracked. It affects both children and adults and most commonly manifests itself on small patches of the body such as on the hands, wrists, insides of the elbows, backs of the knees and the face and scalp, although it can be widespread and visible anywhere. Eczema is considered a long-term condition, known to often come and go. For some their condition will improve and their eczema will disappear completely, often for a long time without a sign, only for it to reappear sometime later.

Why does my skin go red and swell?

When the immune system realises a particular irritant has come in contact with our skin, it sends a large number of white blood cells to the skins surface. These white blood cells cause the blood vessels to open up, quickly dilating them so the white blood cells can gain entry to the tissues; this, however, causes redness to the skin. Often with the dilation or widening of the blood vessels, a little bit of blood and plasma is leaked into the surrounding area, causing swelling.

Why does my skin dry up?

When this inflammation initially occurs, the circulation to the oil glands are affected, so less sebum is produced. With less oil on the skin, the skin loses its ability to retain water and dries out. At the same time, the inflammation stretches your cells, affecting their ability to function, causing them to die quicker and flake off.

Why is my skin so itchy?

When inflammation occurs, histamine gathers affecting our nerve endings, causing us to feel an intense itching.

Types of Eczema

Eczema can be broken down into two types:

Endogenous- caused by internal stimulus via the bloodstream.

Exogenous- (commonly known as contact dermatitis) caused by an external stimulus, such as the skin coming into contact with an irritant which the skin is allergic to. By avoiding the particular irritant that causes this allergic reaction, you should in effect be cured.

Common Irritants

Common irritants to avoid include:

•Detergents (biological)

•Cosmetics

•Soaps

•Rubber

•Dyes

•Yeast

•Nickel

Atopic eczema is often common if there is a family tendency towards it. The exact cause of atopic eczema is unknown, but it's clear it is not down to one single thing, and commonly develops alongside other conditions, such as asthma and hay fever.

Treatments and Remedies

Although there is no cure, many different treatments can be applied to help control and manage the symptoms of eczema.

Topical Corticosteroids

Used to reduce swelling, redness and itching during flare-ups. Corticosteroids (steroids) normally come in the form of creams or ointments and can be applied directly onto the skin as a type of medication. Although there are varying strengths which require prescription you can buy the mildest version of hydrocortisone from your local pharmacy without a prescription. Corticosteroids are designed to reduce inflammation and help reduce itching and irritation.

Self-Preservation Techniques

Try to avoid scratching. Although people scratch because there is an itch, sometimes it can be a habit they have when stressed or tired. If you are prone to scratching, try covering the area with a bandage, as well as focusing on ways to sooth the skin and relax.

Emollients

Moisturising treatments should be used on a daily basis to help combat dry skin.

Anti-Inflammatory Diet

Applying an anti-inflammatory diet:

Essential Fatty acids: Make sure your body receives the right type of essential fatty acids. Omega 3 is known to help retain moisture in the skin, but most importantly acts as an anti-inflammatory. Omega 3 is found in oily fish such as salmon, sardines, mackerel, also flax seeds (linseed if unrefined) and rapeseed oil.

Carotenoids: Increase your intake of carotenoids, they are a powerful antioxidant which will help neutralise free radicals produced by white blood cells. Any good antioxidants will help, but fat-soluble antioxidants, such as carotenoids, are particularly good for penetrating deeper into the skin. These are found in bright fruit or vegetables with an orange colour, like carrots, sweet potatoes and pumpkins.

B-vitamins: Often known as the B-Complex they work together for good skin health. They are known to help regulate the function of skin, normalising the process, helping reduce flakiness and inflammation.

Niacin or Vitamin B3 contributes to the nourishment of hair follicle cells, improving your skins ability to retain moisture, reducing dryness and flakiness. B-vitamins also help utilise fatty acids, helping the body process carbohydrates to produce energy from fat, forming the kind of fat designed in particular that combines with the top layer of dead skin to form a protective barrier, without which the skin would lose its natural moisture. So, if consuming Omega 3, make sure you have a good supply of B-vitamins to take full advantage of the benefits.

It's important to ensure you get a good range of all the B-vitamins in your diet as you need B6 to aid Folic acid (B9) in reducing inflammation in the skin and circulatory system and without B6, B12 can't work to reduce inflammation. Luckily, a lot of foods high in one B vitamin tend to be high in the others, so there is a lot of crossover. However, the following B Vitamins are particularly good for Eczema suffers:

Sources Niacin B3: Meat products (chicken, beef, pork, white fish) potatoes, bread (wholemeal in particular), eggs and instant coffee.

Sources of B6: Turkey, white fish, potatoes, wheat germ, bananas and brussels sprouts.

Sources of B12: Only found in animal products and micro-organisms including yeast, which is why **vegetarians and vegans** need to be more aware of this, actively looking to incorporate this in their diet or via supplements. B12 can be found in Marmite, liver, cheese, milk, eggs, beef and white fish

.

Chapter 17: Psoriasis

Psoriasis affects the speed of skin cell turnover. On average skin, cells take four weeks to travel up through the layers of the skin to the surface, where they shed as dead skin cells. In those who have psoriasis, this happens in less than a week, causing patches of redness with silver coloured flaky scales in the centre. These thick, flaky areas tend to be both dry and itchy. Affecting over 120 million people worldwide, psoriasis is one of the most common autoimmune conditions in the world.

Stress

Unfortunately, no one knows the exact cause for psoriasis, yet psoriasis and stress are considered intricately linked. Although psoriasis has links to genetics, there is a genetic tendency to develop it, environmental factors, such as stress, often trigger it. According to the American

Academy of Dermatology, Vesna Petronic-Rosic, MD, dermatologist and associate professor of medicine at the University of Chicago states "Psoriasis is very stress dependent. It flares very easily when patients are under stress, and it tends to improve when they're relaxed". It is often the case with those that have psoriasis; that their first flare-up will coincide with a stressful time in their life. Unfortunately, psoriasis itself is stressful which seems to compound the problem; therefore, stress management is vital.

'Your immune system responds to injury and infection by sending out chemicals that cause inflammation and help heal a wound. In people with psoriasis, the immune system over-responds—it sends out too many of those chemicals. Setting of an inflammatory process which makes skin cells multiply. It is suspected the immune system responds the same way to mental stress.' * www.psoriasis.org

Everyone is different, but find ways to relax that you enjoy. Take time to relax, be that walks, yoga, seeing friends, exercise, or a nice bath. Should you need to talk to someone about any anxieties, please seek help from friends, family or a professional.

Liver Function

The liver is the major 'filter' of the body. If this vital organ becomes overworked, other organs designed to aid waste elimination, such as the skin, must be more heavily relied upon.

Dr John Pagano, a leading holistic psoriasis researcher, strongly believes that an unhealthy liver plays an active role in the development and recurrence of psoriasis. Therefore, reduced alcohol consumption and a healthy diet will put less stress on the skin. There have also been links associated with 'NAFLD' Non-Alcoholic Fatty Liver Disease, published in the journal 'Gastroenterology Review', which focus on the relationship between Psoriasis and its occurrence and NAFLD. Therefore, any steps to increase liver function can be seen as a positive step:

•Drinking more water

•Reducing Alcohol Consumption

•Herbs such as red clover can be found in teas to aid detox of the liver.

Gut lining

The role of good bacteria in the gut is crucial as various probiotic bacteria maintain the integrity of the gut lining. When the balance of bacteria within the gut is threatened, by things such as overuse of antibiotics or even dietary choices, the ability of the good bacteria to maintain the gut wall lining is reduced and you can get what is commonly called 'Leaky gut syndrome'. LPS (Lipopolysaccharide) a chemical found in a large number of gut bacteria, is leaked out and thereby enters your bloodstream, LPS acts as a power switch to turn on inflammation. Therefore, maintaining good bacteria is important and taking a good probiotic supplement can help.

Anti-Inflammatory Diet

Essential Fatty Acids in particular Omega 3 are anti-inflammatory. Essential Fatty Acids cannot be produced naturally in the body and can only be taken through diet. They help the body produce prostaglandins, an anti-inflammatory compound. Omega 3, in particular, will help reduce redness to the skin, as well as helping to lock moisture in the skin. Omega 3 can be found in oily fish, such as salmon, mackerel, anchovies, as well as flaxseeds, chai seeds, walnuts, fresh basil.

B- Vitamins contribute towards healthy skin function. In particular, Folate which is often marketed interchangeably with folic acid, the synthetic version. Folate is the natural form of vitamin B9, found in a variety of plant and animal foods and helps to regulate skin cell turnover, which in psoriasis sufferers is particularly important, helping to slow the process down. Although found in many foods, it is particularly high in offal and raw green leafy vegetables: like spinach, romaine lettuce, as well as asparagus and broccoli.

For further information on B-Vitamins, please refer to the chapter on Eczema – Anti-inflammatory foods - B Vitamins play an important part in good skin health and the information contained there will be strongly beneficial to psoriasis sufferers as well.

Quercetin belongs to a group of plant pigments called flavonoids, responsible for giving many fruits, flowers, and vegetables their bright colours. Flavonoids, such as Quercetin, are antioxidants. Antioxidants neutralise free radicals, helping to slow down and prevent some of the damage they do to our cells. They also act as a great anti-inflammatory. The University of Maryland Medical Centre has been carrying out test tube trials showing Quercetin to be a powerful antioxidant that *"can also help stabilise the cells that release histamine in the body and thereby have an anti-inflammatory and antihistamine effect." "In test tubes, Quercetin prevents immune cells from releasing histamines, which are chemicals that cause allergic reactions."

However recent results in living studies show that the amount of oxidative benefit is significantly reduced when taken orally, as it has a decreased ability to be absorbed and make contact with living tissues. However, should you wish to increase your intake of flavonoids, in particular, Quercetin, I would suggest upping your intake of citrus fruits, apples, onions, parsley, sage, tea, and berries.

Vitamin A Helps to maintain the healthy function of your outer cells, helping to prevent the silver scales developing. Found in beef, liver, carrots, sweet potato and kale.

Reduce Smoking

Smoking more than 15 cigarettes a day requires the body to spend a lot of time eliminating carcinogens and other by-products of smoking cigarettes. This extra strain means less energy is delivered into healthy skin maintenance. Also, nicotine, especially at this level, is known to reduce the body's ability to absorb Vitamin B12, which as mentioned earlier is vital for regulating skin cell turnover.

Phototherapy

Phototherapy involves subjecting the skin to UV light under medical supervision, utilising select light rays most suitable for treating psoriasis. This is either done at home with a phototherapy unit, at a psoriasis clinic or the doctor's surgery. This is not the same as using sunbeds so, don't get them confused. Using public sunbeds substantially increases the chance of developing melanoma and should not be used as a substitute. Using ultraviolet light can be very effective; however, phototherapy requires consistency for optimum results. If considering this as a course of treatment, please be aware there is still a risk of overexposure to UV light.

Application of Emulsion

Apply an emulsion on a daily basis to regularly rehydrate the skin and help prevent dryness and itchiness.

Corticosteroids

Corticosteroids (steroids) normally in the form of cream and ointment, can be applied directly onto the skin as a type of medication. Although there are varying strengths which require prescription you can buy the mildest version of hydrocortisone from your local pharmacy without a prescription. Corticosteroids are designed to reduce inflammation, itching and irritation.

Coal Tar-based Treatments

Coal tar has been found effective in helping to treat psoriasis; helping to slow down the rapid replacement of skin cells, working towards normalising the skin. Helping to descale and reduce inflammation and itching. Coal tar treatment is particularly popular if suffering from psoriasis of the scalp, nowadays various shampoos are available on the market which can be applied as a special treatment.

Chapter 18:
Rosacea

Rosacea involves a redness of the face. When dilation occurs too frequently, it can cause damage to the blood vessels, resulting in permanent dilation and redness.

Rosacea tends to develop over time, normally starting with a tendency to blush easily, or a more pink overall complexion. Most common is a flush or redness that extends over the nose and cheeks. It is often the case rosacea is ignored by people simply assuming they have a pink skin tone rather than a skin disorder.

As Rosacea often worsens pustules and papules that look like acnes can appear. These will cause redness and the condition can be misidentified. However, a tell-tale sign is that there are no blackheads. Rosacea is not acne and must not be treated like acne, regardless of the pustules and papules that may occur or you risk worsening your skin. This is sometimes followed with dry, flaky patches, yet the 'skin type' can be any, dry, oily or combination. In more serious cases bulbous lobules can appear around the nose area, often followed with visible veining.

For those with rosacea, you should only ever use the most sensitive products, as your skin is one of the more reactive. Knowing the triggers is paramount as it is a condition that will get worse over time, so the less damage to capillaries you do the more chance you have of slowing the process down.

Avoid anything which will cause the blood vessels to dilate further:

•In particular extreme temperature changes, especially when you go from cold to hot.

  o   Avoid standing to close to the stove when cooking.
  o   Avoid hot bath/showers.
  o   Do not use saunas.

•Sun exposure.

•Heavy exercise.

•Excessive alcohol consumption.

•Also avoid rubbing of the skin, as this can cause additional trauma.

With such sensitive skin, make sure any products used on the face are free of skin irritants, focus on a gentle routine, allowing you to maintain optimum skin health.

Common Irritants

Common irritants found in skincare that may affect rosacea sufferers include:

•Alcohol

•Peppermint

•Menthol

•Fragrance

•Witch Hazel

•Eucalyptus

When applying a broad-based sunscreen, please make sure it is a physical sunscreen rather than a chemical sunscreen.

As I mentioned before, there is no official cure and without treatment is likely to get worse over time. Oral and topical antibiotics have been used to treat rosacea, yet there is a growing concern about bacterial resistance with taking antibiotics long term. Treatments vary, from person to person and so do success rates, so it is worth discussing it with a specialist.

As you are most sensitive to small triggers, a small change in diet may have a big impact on your skin.

Anti-Inflammatory Diet

Anti-inflammatory dietary suggestions:

•Avoiding eating spicy foods.

•Drinking alcohol, as this will cause you to flush.

•Be aware of sugars. Sugars are found in so many things, as there is a direct link between an increase in blood sugars and an increase in inflammation, if you have a high sugar diet its worth being aware it could be contributing to inflammation of your skin eliciting your rosacea.

•Please refer to my section on 'Eczema- Anti-Inflammatory Foods' for information on Essential Fatty Acids and B-Vitamins.

•Make sure your diet is packed full of anti-oxidants, particularly those found in fruit and vegetables as these are beneficial for preventing damage to your cells.

Chapter 19:
Dark spots/Age Spots and Pigmentation

Overproduction of melanin causes dark spots/age spots or hyperpigmentation (commonly seen as darkened patches of skin varying in size and colour). There are common types all caused by different factors.

Exposure to UV rays

These sun related dark spots known as Lentigines, are caused by overexposure to UV rays and are common with the majority of people over the age of sixty. Yet if you have been in the sun a lot during your lifetime, you can develop these earlier on.

Incorporating an SPF in your moisturiser or daily application of a sunscreen is a great preventative measure for anybody who wants to reduce the chance of pigmentation occurring as you age. Most people become concerned with pigmentation when it becomes visibly noticeable and suddenly start applying a SPF as a way of trying to prevent it getting worse. Although awareness of SPF is to be praised, you are, yet somewhat too late if your concern is lentigines and their appearance in the first place. The best course of action is to apply daily, to help prevent formation many years later. As it can take years for pigmentation to surface, the earlier you start, the better prevention results you can achieve. The same is true if you want to prevent premature ageing, with sun exposure being one of the most major contributors to premature ageing on the skin.

Nowadays, sunscreen is so readily available in products. It should be easy to find one you can incorporate into your routine, yet for those concerned that an spf may alter the texture of the product in question negatively (which with a good formulation should not be the case) or you have simply found the perfect day cream and the thought of changing it, when your skin is so good, brings you to tears, there are 'city screens'; little gems in my opinion. These products come in the form of a light liquid, more fluid than a lotion, designed to go on top of a moisturiser. Normally incredibly lightweight with a higher SPF. I have a SPF 50, oil-free version, which I apply daily on top of my moisturiser. Great for out and about in town, no need to worry and amazing under makeup.

Remember however for sunbathing or prolonged periods of sun exposure, remember to wear a more resilient sunscreen designed for durability in weather conditions.

Hormone fluctuations

Melasma Pigmentation will form when there are changes to hormone levels, which is why it is commonly found in ladies who are pregnant, as well as those going through menopause, or hormone therapy treatment. Hyperpigmentation causes your skin to become damaged in the same way, as acne or a burn would affect the pigmentation of the skin.

Medication

Dark spots can also be caused by some medications, making the skin more sensitive to the sun and increasing the likely hood of development. While others, unfortunately, can cause dark spots to appear without any sun exposure. If taking medication, do review the description of possible side effects. Those who are suffering from Liver disease, Addison's disease, Pituitary tumours or hemochromatosis are most susceptible.

Although dark spots feel the same as normal skin and are generally harmless, if you have any concerns always visit a doctor as a precaution, to rule out any cancerous growths.

Dark spots can be treated via a medical procedure, medication, or home treatment. Creams and serums are available in your local beauty hall, often claiming to reduce the visibility of dark spots and pigmentation. From my experience they do have an affect skin tone; although visible results are normally more apparent after six months. Although they may not remove entirely remove them, my feedback from customers over the years is that they do appear to fade with use.

Final Thoughts

As you know, your skin is an organ and as with all organs your body functions best when it receives the right nutrients. Although I believe strongly in a good skincare routine, the health of the skin can be aided significantly, by feeding the body with anti-inflammatory foods and a healthy and varied diet. Even a few days of healthy eating can reduce blotchiness in the skin, and calm down inflamed and red skin. This is certainly true in my personal experience. Yet adopt long-term healthy life habits and your skin will glow from within.

Take time to look after yourself, focus on creating time to relax. A lot of skin issues arise from stress, so please prioritise relaxation. DO IT FOR YOU.

Your skin is like a barometer it reflects what is going on internally, mentally, and is subject to external factors. Listen to it. Analyse it. Look after it. You learnt through this book what you need to do to get the best form your skin. Adapt it to your skins ever-changing needs. Your ability to read your skin will make the biggest difference in your ability to treat it.

Enjoy the process of looking after your skin, as you will be doing this for the rest of your life, learn to enjoy it. Think of it as a reward. A bit of your time.

Don't forget to rest; give your body and its largest organ a chance to repair.

Remember long-term consistency is the key. Follow the rules and you can't go wrong. You'll be pleased with your skin and its appearance for many years to come!

Thank you.

Best wishes for your skin

Always

Angela Xx

Thankyou

I just wanted to take a moment to say thank you to some very special people who have helped me in this journey.

Thank you to my good friend, Sarah who took the time out to read this book through, for her honesty and guidance and great grammar, thank you for your time and support. I can't tell you how much it has meant to me. Xx

To my wonderful Dad thank you for always being there to help, thank you for going through this book, and for always being there to offer support, guidance, and your time whenever I have needed it. Mum & Dad, you have always provided me with an environment, where I grew up believing, if I put my mind to something, I could do anything. Thank you. From the bottom of my heart x

To my husband, thank you for being different to everyone else, without whom I wouldn't be the person I am today. Thank you for showing me the world of the self-employed and for showing me courage; in the way you do business. . With all my love. Xx

To the Girls and their partners, of which I am truly blessed. Thank you for always rallying behind me, and for always being supportive. Thank you for sharing this journey with me. I am so lucky to know you all. I love you all x

To Stephen, thank you for inspiring me to write this book, your inspiration to put pen to paper and take charge of my destiny. I will always thank you.

To 'My Ladies', without you where would this book be, you are the inspiration behind this very book.

To you, yes you, thank you so much for purchasing this book and taking the time to read through this book to the very end It means a lot to me personally, so thank you. Best wishes for you and your skin Xx

DISCLAIMER AND LEGAL NOTICES:

This document is geared towards providing exact and reliable information in regards to the topic and issue covered. The publication is sold with the idea that the publisher is not required to render accounting, officially permitted, or otherwise, qualified services. If advice is necessary, legal or professional, a practised individual in the profession should be ordered. This book should in no way be a substitute for not seeking professional help from your local doctor or dermatologist. The material in this publication is provided for educational and informational purposes only and is not intended as medical advice. The information contained in this book should not be used to diagnose or treat any illness, metabolic disorder, disease or health problem.

From a Declaration of Principles which was accepted and approved equally by a Committee of the American Bar Association and a Committee of Publishers' and Associations. In no way is it legal to reproduce, duplicate, or transmit any part of this document in either electronic means or in printed format. Recording of this publication is strictly prohibited and any storage of this document is not allowed unless with written permission from the publisher. All rights reserved.

The information provided herein is stated to be truthful and consistent, in that any liability, in terms of inattention or otherwise, by any usage or abuse of any policies, processes, or directions contained within is the solitary and utter responsibility of the recipient reader. Under no circumstances will any legal responsibility or blame be held against the publisher for any reparation, damages, or monetary loss due to the information herein, either directly or indirectly.

Respective authors own all copyrights not held by the publisher.

The information herein is offered for informational purposes solely and is universal as such. The presentation of the information is without a contract or any type of guarantee assurance.

The trademarks that are used are without any consent, and the publication of the trademark is without permission or backing by the trademark owner. All trademarks and brands within this book are for clarifying purposes only and are the owned by the owners themselves, not affiliated with this document.

www.ingramcontent.com/pod-product-compliance
Lightning Source LLC
Chambersburg PA
CBHW072247260726
48659CB00004BA/1469